# Diabetes Diet Options

## What to Eat, When to Eat
## and
## How to Regain Your Health

*Nick –*
*To your health!*
*Marian Hays*

Marian Hays

Marian Hays

# TABLE OF CONTENTS

## RAVE REVIEWS

### *Great Resource for Diabetics and Family Members*

*"This book is a great resource for anyone who wants to know more about their diet options as a diabetic, or anyone who has a diabetic family member and needs to know better how to prepare meals and plan what foods to serve. She even covers vegetarian options. There is a lot of important information in this book that no diabetic should be without."*    *Joanna Martin*

### *This Book is a Must for Diabetics*

*"This book is an encyclopedia of good information for those with diabetes, or for those with family members wanting to learn more about diabetes. Presented in an easy to read and therefore easy to understand style, I found it has something for everyone. For those wanting to control their symptoms in as natural a way as possible through good food choices, through to diabetics who are vegetarians. Big news to me was having a good amount of good carbs in your body, and those foods to avoid with bad carbs. A great book, thank you to the author."* *Dailyreader*

# DEDICATION

This book is dedicated to my husband, Mike, who has cheered me on and encouraged me to share my research and insights. While we're very different, we've learned to allow those differences to make each of us better.

He'll tell you that the information I researched saved his life. Actually, it was also the choices he made with the information. Besides the right foods, he believes there are two basics that will make a quality of life difference: portion size and exercise. He says his first exercise was pushing away from the table.

When I originally wrote this book, we were celebrating our 34th anniversary. We've now passed the 38-year mark.

Marian Hays

# INTRODUCTION

On that Friday in August, 2009, my husband went for a checkup and blood test, and the internist recommended a heart specialist for additional tests. He scheduled 4 tests over a period of a month, beginning the following Monday.

While he was at his first heart appointment, the internist's office called with his diagnosis of type 2 diabetes. I was stunned. Meanwhile the heart doctor was changing next week's appointment to the next day. On Tuesday, the doctor moved the third test to Wednesday, after which he advised my husband that he needed an angioplasty procedure: Would you like that on Thursday or Friday? Wake up call!

Friday morning the surgeon inserted a catheter and camera through his vein and into his heart. Four stints were positioned to open blockages of 70%, 80%, 90% and 100% (open the width of a human hair). A friend who'd had the same procedure told me the first words he'd say would be how much better he felt already. Indeed, those were his exact first words.

We found ourselves facing life changing choices. We were fortunate. But it sent us on a search for proper nutrition, what foods he could and should eat, what exercise was best, and what supplements to take. In addition to an ominous list of prescription meds.

I love to research and he was motivated to follow the steps necessary to control Type 2 diabetes and bring his blood sugar numbers back into a safe range. We got here through neglect of proper nutrition and exercise. Yet we're so blessed to discover it before it resulted in a life-threatening heart attack. My husband has learned much of this through my research, without him having to sift through it all on his own. He's cool with that.

I shared with a friend what a "good sport" he was to go cold turkey on certain foods, to read product labels, and to basically follow what I'd researched.  She laughed, held out both hands like she was weighing options, and said, "Good sport, die, good sport, die… yes, I think good sport was the right choice."

He's been under a doctor's care with regular checkups. Our initial goal was to get his numbers "under control" so that he could be weaned off the numerous meds he takes. His original doctor wasn't particularly interested in that, so he researched doctors and found one more interested in getting him healthy and reducing or removing at least some of the meds.  I have a personal goal of having the doctors totally amazed at his results and pronouncing him med-free. Healing *can* happen!

I've been an advocate for healthy eating for some time, but haven't always followed through. I think green smoothies are great, but my Good Sport hasn't ventured that far yet. No problem. There are lots of other choices.

In my research, I learned positive and negative things about the foods we find in grocery stores and restaurants. We started our journey together… if he couldn't eat dessert, I skipped it too. We made great progress. Then I got a bit sloppy in our food habits, yielding to his desire for "forbidden" foods. What he did, I did. Occasional sugar free cheesecake, sweet potato fries? Oops… we started gaining weight again. But he kept his numbers in the safe range.

We're back on track and able to make even better strides. Nothing is a straight line to the top, but has zigs and zags along the way. The idea is to catch that zag soon enough to keep the line only slightly curvy instead of wild swings.

Whether you've just been diagnosed or have lived with diabetes for some time, here are some basic facts and guidelines you should know, served up in a fast and easy to consume format. I encourage you to use it in determining your approach to better health. Consider it a Quick Start Guide.

You do have options. Be proactive. Live long and prosper.

# SECTION 1 - DIABETES BASIC INFORMATION

## WHAT IS DIABETES?

In 2012, diabetes was the seventh leading cause of death in the United States. Even more chilling, it is the first leading cause of death for children. The rising rates of obesity in this country have also led to rising rates of Type 2 diabetes. Today, one in 11 adults is afflicted with the disease. Over 29 million people have the disorder, with 8 million of them walking around undiagnosed and unaware of their sensitive insulin condition.

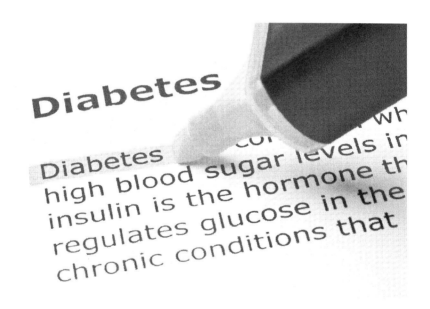

Diabetes results when a person has high blood sugar either because the pancreas doesn't produce enough insulin or because the cells do not respond to the insulin that is produced. This high blood sugar produces diabetic symptoms including frequent urination, increased thirst, and increased hunger, feeling tired, edgy, or sick to the stomach, blurred vision, or tingling or loss of feeling in the hands.

Type 1 diabetes results from the body's failure to produce insulin, and currently requires the person to inject insulin or wear an insulin pump.

Type 2 diabetes is the most common type, and results from insulin resistance, a condition in which cells fail to use insulin properly, sometimes combined with an absolute insulin deficiency. Frequently Type 2 diabetics have a relatively reduced insulin secretion.

The term "insulin dependent" was created in the 1950s on the assumption that muscle and fat require insulin to take up glucose (created by eating high carbohydrate and sugary foods). Current studies show that many different things in the body transport glucose. Cells require glucose for their cell respiration process. The body makes sure that the cells receive that, no matter how much insulin in present. However, insulin is the key that unlocks the cells to allow the proper absorption of nutrients and flushing out the toxins.

Medications are prescribed to improve insulin sensitivity or reduce glucose production by the liver. Unfortunately, some studies show that the meds to help the diabetes can also negatively affect the heart. They should be monitored by your physician on a regular basis. Be sure to discuss possible side effects.

Working with your diabetes diagnosis through diet gives your body a more natural chance of stabilizing and helping you to control your blood sugar, blood pressure, and the many numbers used to see how you're maintaining a healthier state. If medication has been prescribed, it's advisable to keep taking it while you work with your diet. Then you and your physician can work together to see if you can have lower dosages of meds or have some eliminated altogether.

The third main form, gestational diabetes occurs when pregnant women without a previous diagnosis of diabetes develop a high blood glucose level. It may precede development of type 2 diabetes, although it usually reverses after delivery.

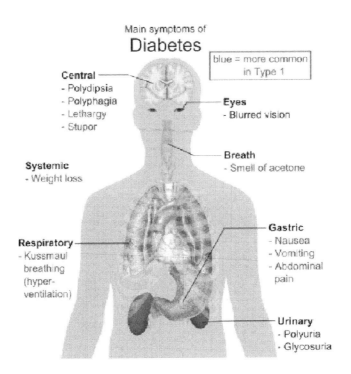

Main symptoms of
## Diabetes

blue = more common in Type 1

**Central**
- Polydipsia
- Polyphagia
- Lethargy
- Stupor

**Eyes**
- Blurred vision

**Breath**
- Smell of acetone

**Systemic**
- Weight loss

**Respiratory**
- Kussmaul
  breathing
  (hyper-
  ventilation)

**Gastric**
- Nausea
- Vomiting
- Abdominal
  pain

**Urinary**
- Polyuria
- Glycosuria

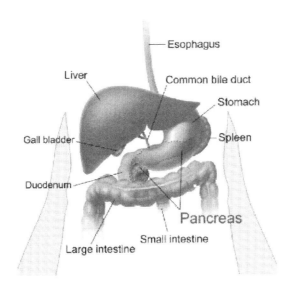

Esophagus

Liver

Common bile duct

Stomach

Gall bladder

Spleen

Duodenum

Pancreas

Large intestine

Small intestine

## DIABETES COMPLICATIONS: BAD NEWS / GOOD NEWS

Untreated, your diabetes can cause many complications. Properly treated you may avoid or slow down adverse conditions. You should be aware of potential complications so you can proactively choose a healthier lifestyle. I'm assuming your goal is a high quality and longer life.

All forms of diabetes increase the risk of long-term complications. Untreated, diabetes can cause several complications. Regrettably, some of the complications may already be occurring when you get your diagnosis, simply because diabetes can go unrecognized and, therefore, untreated for years. Occasionally the treatment for another condition, such as heart issues or vision loss, may be the trigger in discovering that you have diabetes.

These complications are far less common and less severe in people who have well-managed blood sugar levels. Adequate treatment of diabetes is, therefore, very important, as well as blood pressure control and lifestyle factors such as not smoking and maintaining a healthy body weight.

Acute complications include diabetic coma (ketoacidosis and nonketotic hyperosmolar). Insulin is the "key" to open your blood cells to receive and process glucose and produce energy.

Because your cells have become insulin resistant (type 2) or your body isn't producing insulin (type 1), the cells are locked, leaving glucose in the bloodstream. The body continues to burn fat, but this causes the liver to make more and more ketones and ketoacids. The increasing levels make the blood highly acidic, which becomes an emergency that requires immediate medical attention.

Serious long-term complications include cardiovascular disease, chronic renal failure, and diabetic retinopathy (retinal damage). These typically develop after 10–20 years, but may be the first symptom in those who have otherwise not received a diabetic diagnosis sooner.

The major long-term complications relate to damage to blood vessels. Diabetes doubles the risk of cardiovascular disease. The main "macrovascular" diseases (related to atherosclerosis of larger arteries) are ischemic heart disease (angina and myocardial infarction), stroke and peripheral vascular disease.

Diabetes also damages the capillaries (causes microangiopathy). Diabetic retinopathy, which affects blood vessel formation in the retina of the eye, can lead to visual symptoms including reduced vision and, potentially, blindness. A friend diagnosed with diabetes a few years ago, took his prescription meds, but paid no attention to diet and lifestyle.

He was recently declared legally blind, totally affecting his ability to do his job.

Diabetic nephropathy, the impact of diabetes on the kidneys, can lead to scarring changes in the kidney tissue, loss of small or progressively larger amounts of protein in the urine, and eventually chronic kidney disease requiring dialysis.

Another risk is diabetic neuropathy, the impact of diabetes on the nervous system - most commonly causing numbness, tingling and pain in the feet, and also increasing the risk of skin damage due to altered sensation. Together with vascular disease in the legs, neuropathy contributes to the risk of diabetes-related foot problems (such as diabetic foot ulcers) that can be difficult to treat and occasionally requires amputation. Also, proximal diabetic neuropathy causes painful muscle wasting and weakness.

OK, that was the technical and gloomy information. However, it's important to understand how your body responds to changes in your pancreas function.

## THERE IS HOPE

Management of the disease concentrates on keeping blood sugar levels as close to normal as possible, without causing hypoglycemia. This can usually be accomplished with diet, exercise, and use of appropriate medications (insulin in the case of type 1 diabetes; oral medications and possibly insulin in type 2 diabetes).

You can start now to align your body to absorb what it needs, understand what is happening on the inside, and prevent degenerative progression. You don't have to accept a fatal result or give up without your best effort to reverse or stop the progress.

## DIABETES DIETS AND SUPPLEMENTS

You have several diabetic diet options. Read through them, see how you can fit them into your lifestyle or decide how you need to alter your lifestyle to live a longer, healthier one.

Choose whole foods for their nutritional value, especially since they will contain a variety of nutrients. Unfortunately, much of our foods are over-processed and insufficient so supplements are advisable.

Many studies in recent years have proven that antioxidants help prevent diabetic complications, especially neuropathy and retinopathy. Most people know what they do and why we need them, but questions remain, like how much and which ones.

Antioxidant experts call diabetes a "free radical disease." People with diabetes use up their antioxidant stores more quickly, so their requirements are actually higher. This is because diabetes creates more free radicals, and free radicals use up the vitamins, therefore you need more.

Vitamins are also flushed through a diabetic's body at an alarming rate. Therefore, making sure you take proper dosages of necessary vitamins gives your body the best possible chance for absorbing what you need.

Be sure to take a good multivitamin (there are special diabetic packs available) because you need the vitamins, and you simply aren't going to get enough through food alone. This may be true for all of us with the highly-processed foods we eat, but it's much more so for the diabetic.

One of the often overlooked but very important vitamin is Vitamin D, known as the sunshine vitamin. It improves insulin sensitivity by up to 60%, according to extensive research. Those are better numbers than the diabetic drug metformin. It also has been shown to lesson complications of cardiovascular disease. Some foods high in Vitamin D include liver (I know, everyone's favorite), wild salmon, shrimp, cod, eggs and milk, pus red, yellow and orange fruits and vegetables and dark green leafy vegetables. Since it is sometimes overlooked in the typical vitamin packs, you might want to ask your physician to check your Vitamin D.

## THE GLYCEMIC INDEX

The Glycemic Index assigns foods a ranking from 1-100 that indicates its affect on blood sugar levels. This can take some of the guess work out of meal planning and what foods to eat.

Foods that have a low Glycemic Index (GI) value mean they will take a longer time to affect your blood sugars. Foods that have a higher value will act quicker to raise blood sugars. Obviously, lower is better.

Unfortunately, just using the Glycemic Index to decide what to eat or avoid isn't enough. Just because a food has a low GI doesn't mean it has the nutrition we need. Some foods on the higher end of the scale can be better because of the nutritional value. Also, not all foods are listed.

It is, however, an important piece of information as you plan a proper diet for yourself. And planning is critical.

You can find glycemic index charts online, and see GI for your favorite foods. If you want even more information on how to incorporate the GI diet with your current meal plan, consult with your dietician or a diabetes educator.

## BENEFITS OF A HEALTHY DIABETIC DIET

Eating well can help control your diabetes and prolong your life expectancy.

Benefits of eating a healthy diet are for everyone, but for a diabetic there can be even more reasons to follow a nutritious meal plan. Keeping a stable blood glucose level is the biggest reason for a diabetic to follow a diabetic diet. It takes commitment and patience to stick with planning all your meals each week. But the more that's done, the easier it will become.

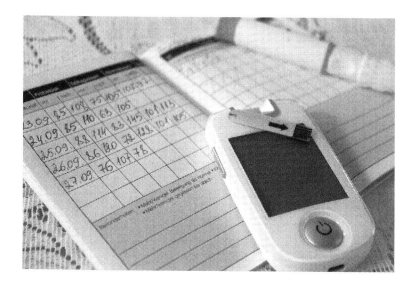

If one member of your family is better at this than you are, encourage their support in getting the meal plans working.

Some families discover this is a perfect opportunity for all family members to make more healthy food choices. This may also prevent others from some day having the same diagnosis of diabetes. Be aware that the tendency to develop diabetes is considered hereditary.

Another benefit of eating a healthy diabetic diet is reducing the amount of insulin that is needed. By eating good carbohydrate choices and lean meats you will lower the insulin requirements for your body. All foods you eat affect your blood sugars and when you do not choose the best foods for your body, it will need more insulin to process them. In addition to extra insulin requirements, you will suffer from high blood sugars, also known as hyperglycemia. This condition can have serious long-term effects on your body and its organs.

By continuing with a healthy diet and combining it with regular exercise you can also lose any excess body weight. This, too, is good for your insulin requirements and blood glucose levels. By incorporating exercise into your daily routine, you can give your body's metabolism a boost and help it process the foods you're eating. When the foods you take in are healthy choices, your body is going to function better.

If you do not follow a healthy diet, you can suffer from:

* Low blood sugar from not eating enough – hyperglycemia

* High blood sugar from eating too much or eating the wrong foods – hypoglycemia

* Weight gain and, in turn, increase your daily insulin requirement

* Lack of energy needed to exercise on a regular basis

* Other more serious side effects of disease progression, affecting limbs, eyes and more (see Complications)

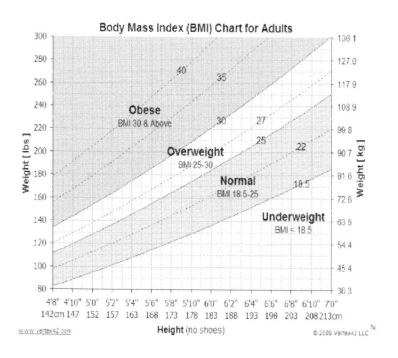

## THE ROLE OF FIBER

The role of fiber in healthy diets is very important. It aids in digestion and keeps your colon and other organs healthy and functioning properly. It's also an important element that should be a large part of any diabetic's diet. You will reap many benefits by including fiber in your diet. If you're pre-diabetic, it can assist in delaying or avoiding a diagnosis of diabetes. If you're already diabetic, it can help keep your blood glucose under control.

Fiber will keep you feeling fuller longer. It slows the conversion of carbohydrates in your body which in turn can keep your blood sugars stable. The type of fiber that a diabetic needs to eat to gain these benefits is soluble fiber (dissolves in water). Some good sources of soluble fiber include:

* Choosing sprouted or whole grain products instead of white (flour, breads, and cereals)
* Eating fresh fruit and vegetables instead of processed or drinking them in liquid form
* Beans - use dried beans in your favorite recipes like chili for a wholesome, high-fiber meal

To ensure that you are getting the most benefit from eating increased amount of fiber, make sure that you are drinking at least eight glasses of water a day (or four 16-ounce water bottles). Fiber dissolves in water and you need to stay hydrated for it to work properly. If this seems like "too much" then drink as much as possible, consistently working toward the magic 64-ounce mark. If others can do it, so can you!

If you're on the carbohydrate counting diet and are using 15 grams of carbohydrates as one serving, you can increase the amount you're eating if that item has high-fiber content. Subtract the number of grams of fiber in a serving from the number of carbohydrates. For instance, if you are eating an item that has 20 grams of carbohydrates (which is over the single serving limit) but it has five grams of fiber, you can subtract the five from the twenty and it now only counts as a 15-gram serving.

## PROTEIN'S EFFECT ON BLOOD SUGAR LEVELS

Much the same as fiber, eating quality protein with your snacks and meals can have a positive effect on your blood sugar levels. By combining protein and carbohydrates you will slow the digestion of the carbohydrates in your body. This slowing down will prevent your blood sugar from spiking as the result of too many carbohydrates in your system.

This does not mean that you should eat more protein than is recommended in one meal. Doing so can lead to other problems down the road. As a diabetic, skipping protein in your diet is not a good idea. For vegetarians or diabetics who usually don't eat a lot of protein, it's important to find a source that can be consumed on a regular basis.

There are many sources of high-quality protein that don't include animal meats.

* Tofu is a source of protein that can be prepared in a variety of ways including dessert tofu
* Nuts are an excellent source of protein but can be high in fat too. Read nutrition labels and enjoy in moderation
* Seeds such as flax, pumpkin, and sunflower can be eaten as a source of protein
* Beans and other members of the legume family. There are

many ways to prepare beans, from chili to cold salads

* Protein powders are available to sprinkle on cereals or to make into shakes for drinking

* Fish. Be aware that large fish contain high levels of mercury and should only be eaten once or twice per week

When making protein choices, go for a lean cut whenever possible. Even though protein has a positive effect on blood sugars, excessive fat can cancel out the benefit and turn it into a health risk.

## Consistency and Variety

There are several diets especially geared for people with diabetes. Or you can learn what foods are best at controlling your sugar levels, and what foods to avoid, thereby creating your own eating plan. Whatever you choose, it doesn't have to be boring or restrictive.

You didn't get to this diagnosis overnight and without eating foods that haven't served you well. However, if you choose well now, and stick with it, you should be able to master the numbers and extend your life.

Being consistent and having variety in your diet at the same time is possible! The consistency comes with specific meal times and the size servings from different food groups. And the variety refers to trying as many different foods in the food groups as you can.

It can be easy to find a few meals that work well with your blood sugars and are easy to prepare and just stick with them. You are more than likely to get bored with this, and you probably aren't getting all the nutrients you need from a repetitive set amount of foods.

You have a lot of room for flexibility. You can combine different foods together for something new or try foods you have never had before. You can meet with your dietician to get additional ideas for recipes and other foods that you can eat to add more variety to your diet.

There will be times that you try a new food and your blood sugars are higher as a result. If this is the case, think back about anything else that you did differently that day such as less activity or taking your insulin (if you are Type I) later than usual. If the new food is the only change you experienced, talk to your dietician. You may be able to prepare the food differently or eat it with something else, or you may have to avoid that food if it doesn't work for your diabetic diet. Keeping a food diary, such as this book's companion Diabetes Journal, is a good idea as you start your journey to regaining health.

Just because you have diabetes doesn't mean that you can't be adventurous and try something new, just do it at regular meal times and within the recommended portion sizes. The stronger your resolve, the better your results.

# SECTION 2 – DIABETES NUTRITION: WHAT TO EAT

## 1) CARBOHYDRATE COUNTING

Carbohydrates have a very big impact on blood glucose levels as they're converted to sugar by the body in the process of turning the food into energy. Too many carbohydrate servings can increase blood sugar levels. It's important for a diabetic to control the number of carbohydrates that are eaten at each meal and balance the carbohydrates with protein while limiting fat intake.

In this type of meal plan, foods are grouped into three different categories: carbohydrates, proteins, and fats. Most foods that you eat contain carbohydrates and this will be the largest food group. Foods in this group include:

* Grains - breads, crackers, rice, cereal, pasta
* Dairy - milk, yogurt
* Vegetables that are considered starchy - corn, peas, and potatoes
* The rest of the vegetable family
* Fruit, including fruit juices (which may also be high in sugar)
* Desserts and other treats – chosen in limited amounts

This diet will require you to measure your foods for serving sizes and read food labels to determine how many carbohydrate servings it has.

It is standard to consider 15 grams of carbohydrates as one serving. For instance, if you're having crackers as a snack and are allowed one serving of carbohydrates you would look at the food label to figure out how many crackers you can have. If the serving size is 20 crackers and that equals 30 grams of carbohydrates, for a diabetic that would be considered two servings. In this example, you would half the serving size and eat 10 crackers to equal 15 grams of carbohydrates.

After some time and experience you'll become adept at counting carbohydrates and knowing what foods work well with your blood glucose levels and what ones don't. No two diabetics respond the same way to every food. You will need to learn what your own ideal diabetic diet is.

## BENEFITS OF THE CARBOHYDRATE COUNTING DIET

As stated, the carbohydrate counting diet groups foods into carbohydrates, proteins, and fats. Your dietician or physician will provide you with the number of carbohydrates you can have in a day and how that is divided up among your meals and snacks. He or she will also educate you on how you can determine the number of carbohydrates in some of your favorite foods by reading food labels.

The biggest benefit of the carbohydrate counting diet is that it does not eliminate any foods. Diabetics can choose any food they wish to eat as long as they only eat enough of it to meet their carbohydrate needs and no more. The trick is to choose wholesome foods that will fill you up longer. The same amounts of carbohydrates that are in a small handful of potato chips are not equal to the two slices of bread you can have instead. But it is nice to know that if you really want to - once in awhile - you can treat yourself.

Another benefit is keeping a consistent amount of carbohydrates in your body. This can help regulate your insulin needs and control. If your body has the same amount of carbohydrates to process at the same times each day it will be beneficial to your health and blood glucose readings.

When you choose a carbohydrate counting diet, it is important to make sure you are doing it correctly. If you don't, you can eat too much or too little and both situations can be detrimental to your health. Have a dietician teach you how to properly count carbohydrates and closely monitor your blood sugar levels to make sure the diet it working for you.

As with any new diet, give it time for you to adjust and learn how to plan your meals properly.

## GOOD CARBOHYDRATES AND BAD CARBOHYDRATES

Diabetic diets and diabetic meal planning are often centered around carbohydrate intake. This is the amount you can have and when you should have them. This is because they play such a crucial role in managing blood sugars. Too many carbohydrates or the wrong kind can cause high blood sugars. Not enough carbohydrates can cause low blood sugars or hypoglycemia.

It is recommended that carbohydrates make up about 40% of your daily calories, but not all carbohydrates are created equal. You also need to pay attention to fat and sugar content.

Here are some healthier carbohydrate choices:

* Whole grain cereals
* Whole wheat breads and rolls
* Brown rice
* Whole wheat crackers
* Raw or lightly steamed fruits and vegetables
* Whole wheat pita pockets or wraps

(Note: Whole wheat is not as healthy as it was previously. But it's still better than white breads.)

Carbohydrate choices to avoid:

* Potato chips
* White bread
* White rice
* Processed foods
* Cookies
* Easy to eat snacks

Carbohydrates are an essential part of every diet but make sure you are including the right kinds in yours. Good carbohydrates will fill you up and not create a sudden spike in your blood sugars. Bad carbohydrates are usually over-processed, create high blood sugars, create obesity and are high in sodium. (Note: while you need to restrict salt or sodium intake, you will benefit by choosing low sodium foods and using a salt high in minerals. Look for pink Himalayan salt in the organic or health food aisles of your grocery store, or order online.)

It's important to fill your body with high-quality choices. Choose carbohydrates that provide energy and not weight gain. The less processed or refined a carbohydrate is the better it is going to be for you. Even when baking, choose unbleached whole grain flour. It doesn't make a big difference in taste but it does in the quality of carbohydrate it creates. Try whole grain flour in pancakes. Ezekiel bread made of sprouted grains is a great healthier alternative. You'll find this in the frozen foods section, sometimes with organic items.

Marian Hays

## 2) THE EXCHANGE DIET

The exchange diet is one that allows you to choose the foods you eat from each of the six food groups based on portion sizes. When you begin eating with this diet, it may seem like a lot of work, but as you get used to the portions sizes and the common substitutions that you make, it will get easier.

One of the benefits of the exchange diet it the flexibility you have in your meal planning. If you are eating the correct number of exchanges from each food group, you will maintain better control of your blood glucose levels.

The exchange diet might be for you if you get bored quite easily with eating the same foods day in and day out. There are endless possibilities to combine foods differently at meal times. You can have broccoli for dinner three nights in a row but make it a completely different meal each time. One night you can have one small potato, ½ cup of steamed broccoli and a one ounce pork chop; the second night have ½ cup of cooked pasta tossed with ½ cup of broccoli and one ounce of cooked chicken; and the third night try 1/3 cup of brown rice mixed with ½ cup of broccoli and one ounce of lean beef.

The exchange diet also takes the guess work out of meal planning. It is laid out in a very straight forward and easy to understand manner. If there are foods that you cannot find on the exchange list given to you by your dietician, call and find out which group it belongs to and what a proper portion size is.

At first you should weigh and measure your foods to ensure you are using the proper amounts but as time passes you will be able to do this by sight.

## 3) A DIABETIC DIET FOR VEGETARIANS

If you're a vegetarian who has been diagnosed with diabetes, you can still maintain your diabetic diet. In some cases, a vegetarian diet may be a healthy way to keep your blood glucose levels stable if you are eating lean high-quality proteins and are following other rules for eating as a diabetic.

A lot of vegans and vegetarians eat a larger amount of fruits and vegetables in a day than a non-vegetarian, and their fiber intake is much higher too. An increased amount of fiber in a diabetic's diet can help blood sugars because it slows down the process of the body digesting carbohydrates. A vegetarian's diet is usually lower in cholesterol, as well, and that can help ward off cardiovascular disease including heart attacks and strokes.

If you're considering a switch to a vegetarian diet, some of the benefits you might derive include a higher rate of weight loss and better blood sugar readings. This is dependent on the types of vegetarian meals you choose as some meatless meals can be just as fattening as ones that contain meat.

Speak to your doctor and dietician before making the switch. You will need information on how to transition yourself to your new diet. You will also get a list of meat alternatives you should eat to get enough protein in a day. These can include tofu, nuts, eggs, and seeds.

As with any change, once you switch to a vegetarian diet, give yourself and your body time to adjust. There are many recipes and ideas for vegetarian dishes and you will find a lot of variety and flexibility in the meals that you prepare. Check your blood sugars frequently to make sure your blood glucose levels remain stable during the change.

## THREE HEALTH ADVANTAGES OF A VEGETARIAN DIET

While some people lament nutritional disadvantages of a poorly planned vegetarian diet, few stress the health advantages of adopting a vegetarian or vegan diet.

One major advantage of a vegetarian diet is increased heart health. Vegetarians, on average, consume more nuts (often as a supplemental form of protein). Nuts contain "good" fats, such as omega-3 and omega-6. This promotes good heart health by reducing "bad" cholesterol and unclogging arteries.

In addition to nuts, vegetarians also consume more soy milk (often to replace milk), which reduces "bad" cholesterol and has been linked to good heart health. Almond and coconut milks are also good choices, especially if you want to avoid dairy.

Increased skin health is a second major advantage vegetarians enjoy. In addition to consuming larger quantities of nuts (which contain healthful oils), vegetarians tend to consume more fruit and vegetables, which are rich in essential vitamins, including A and E, which are linked to good skin health. Fruits and vegetables also contain high amounts of fiber, which helps flush toxins out of the body, further contributing to better skin health.

A third health advantage is an increased natural consumption of antioxidants. Antioxidants are foods that help prevent cancer by destroying free radicals. Vitamin C and Vitamin E, two strong antioxidants, are commonly found in vegetarian meals.

Vitamin C can be found in berries, tomatoes, citrus fruit, kale, kiwis, asparagus, and peppers.

Vitamin E can be found in wheat germ, seed oils, walnuts, almonds, and brown rice - all foods that are commonly a part of a well-balanced vegetarian diet.

Vitamin D is found in red, yellow and orange fruits and vegetables and dark green leafy vegetables.

So, what does this mean for you as a prospective vegetarian? Not only can a vegetarian diet be nutritionally sufficient, but it can also affect better skin health, prevent cancer, and increase your heart health.

## 4) THE THERAPEUTIC LIFESTYLE CHANGES (TLC) DIET

The TLC diet was developed with more than diabetics in mind. It is a diet recommended to people with high cholesterol, heart, or other cardiovascular diseases and those that have been diagnosed with diabetes.

This diet consists of a set of guidelines that provide percentage ranges of what a patient should eat from each food group. The aim is to provide flexibility in choices while ensuring that the choices made are helpful to the condition that is being treated. In the beginning, it's a good idea to partner with a dietician to ensure the calculations that you are making are accurate and that you are making the best food choice decisions.

The TLC diet provides the following eating guidelines:

* The total amount of fat that is eaten in a day should add up to less than 25-35% of the calories that are consumed
* Of the 25-35% fat intake it should be broken down into the following categories: less than 7% saturated; less than 20% monounsaturated; 10% polyunsaturated
* 50-60% of a day's worth of calories should be derived from carbohydrates
* Eat at least 20-30 grams of high-quality fiber each day

* The protein consumed should equal 15-20% of the calories for the day
* Cholesterol should be limited and kept under 200 mg per day

As the diet is a set of guidelines that do not include the calculations necessary to determine if you are meeting the requirements, you should book an appointment with a dietician to understand what you need to do. Once you have been shown how to make the calculations and have been given a sample meal plan you can use those as a template to create many variations of the TLC diet. You can also glean much of this information by reading the food labels on packages.

## 5) DANIEL DIET - ELIMINATING CERTAIN FOODS FOR A PERIOD OF TIME

The Daniel Diet is not a fad diet to lose weight. The Daniel diet is based on a verse from the Bible.

Daniel 1:18 says, "Daniel purposed in his heart that he would not defile himself" with the types of foods being offered to the Hebrews living in exile. The Babylonians ate rich foods lacking nutrition that included non-kosher food, wine, foods offered to idols. Instead Daniel requested a diet focused on healthy foods. The Babylonians were concerned that the young Hebrews choosing to eliminate the rich foods would lead them to become weak and sickly, and therefore unable to work. The opposite was true, as the young Hebrews were stronger and healthier after the test period.

According to the modern-day Daniel fast, you should specifically avoid meat, white flour or white rice, fried foods, caffeine, carbonated beverages (including diet soda), alcohol, foods with any preservatives or additives, refined sugar, high fructose corn syrup, chemical sugar substitutes like Equal, and margarine, shortening or any product with animal fats.

Instead, you are allowed to eat whole grains, legumes, fruits, vegetables, seeds, nuts, and water, fruit juices and vegetable juices.

If you're following this diet for the spiritual reasons as well as the health benefits, prepare through prayer. Make a commitment to stay on the diet for a specified period. You may want to share your commitment with family, friends, and faith partners.

You can also prepare yourself physically for the diet. If you're addicted to caffeine, it is a good idea to wean yourself from coffee or soda for two weeks before starting the Daniel diet. Also, begin reducing meat consumption ahead of time so that this is not a shock to your system.

The length of time you stay on the Daniel Diet depends on you. Some people make a commitment to continue their new food choices for the rest of their lives. Some fast as part of a church-wide program, or for 40 days of Lent. However, you can do the Daniel fast for as little as 7 days and see results. Some people maintain a one day a week fast.

Whether you choose this diet strictly for the nutritional value, or for the full spiritual process, here are some tips to help you be successful on the Daniel Diet.

* Be specific about the number of days on the diet.

* Use your external discipline to reflect your internal desire.

* Pray for guidance about food's role in your physical health.

* Use your fast as an unspoken testimony to others

* Use your fast to learn the effects of the food you eat on your body.

* Give praise to God for whatever successes you have on the Daniel Diet.

Marian Hays

## 6) DIABETES AND THE pH MIRACLE DIET

Type 2 diabetes goes hand in hand with increased aging, obesity, poor nutrition, high stress, and physical inactivity. Less well known is the fact that these conditions can be traced back to one source, namely, high acidity. Over-acid lifestyles and food choices have negative impacts on health, which is shown by the rapidly increasing diabetes rates in the country.

Diabetes has been recognized as a disease for thousands of years, but only in the past few decades that it's become an epidemic. Many people believe that obesity is the cause of diabetes. However, obesity is a result of increased consumption of carbohydrates and sugars. Empty calories, such as alcohol, contribute no nutritional value and are only converted to fat.

The high rate of consumption of these products (which are made from the acidifying foods of sugar and processed wheat) leads to high acidity in the body. The body attempts to deal with the increase of waste acids by using fat to neutralize the acid. The fat is then stored as a safeguard for the cells in the body. It's not unlike a grain of sand in an oyster, except the oyster produces a coating of pearl around the grain of sand to protect itself, whereas the human body adds a coating of fat to prevent the acid from harming us.

Insulin resistance, which is a precursor to Type 2 diabetes, is brought on through a highly acidic lifestyle and acidic food choices. It occurs in the liver, muscles, and fat cells. Excess caffeine, chocolate, sugar, and carbohydrates stimulate these bodily organs and tissues. As the body is stimulated, the cells begin to release their glucose and this leads to the elevated levels of blood sugar that people see when they do blood sugar testing.

The body cells are disorganized, and the highly acidic state can lead to a host of problems overtime including premature aging, high blood pressure, inhibition of the release of glycogen from the liver, and the inhibition of the burning of fat.

Over stimulation of the bodily tissues through acidic foods can cause a lot of damage, and Type 2 diabetes is just a symptom of an acidic lifestyle. When the liver must work overtime to handle the increased glucose, the blood becomes highly acidic and can result in diabetic coma.

To bring the body back into balance, you must include alkalizing green vegetables, green drinks, and good fats in your diet. Plant proteins from grains and legumes also help restore the body's previous homeostasis. The pH miracle diet includes a balanced plan for eating with your body, instead of against it. With the application of the principles of the diet, controlling and preventing diabetes is a simple matter of alkalized eating and living.

The pH miracle diet has similarities with the vegetarian diet as much of those foods are alkaline forming rather than acidic.

Disease simply doesn't thrive in an alkaline body, while acidic foods give disease such as cancer and diabetes a feeding ground to grow and destroy their host bodies. An alkaline body also puts less stress on the pancreas and creates the most favorable environment for healing.

**Choosing alkaline foods, regardless of the diet you choose, may be one of the most important adjustments you can make.**

Some grocery stores are beginning to carry alkaline water. Unlike other bottled waters, which are acidic to your body, the alkaline water increases your alkalinity and improves your overall health.

## 7) NUTRIMOST DIET

Being overweight often leads to diabetes (and other ailments) and becomes a vicious cycle as the diabetes then contributes to weight gain. Finding the right diet to maintain a healthy weight as well as work to control your diagnosis becomes far more important. If weight has ever been an issue for you, this diet may be a good alignment.

Many nutritional diets are simply personal preference, but this is highly targeted to personal results in regaining your health.

Less well known but of unique value to diabetics is the NutriMost Diet Plan. Known for success rates of 20-45 pounds lost in a mere 40 days, the focus is on overall health, not simply weight loss. It's backed with scientific research and doctor supervision. Originally created with body healing in mind, the weight loss success rates made it a popular weight loss program. It maximizes health benefits as you lose harmful fat.

It focuses on healthy natural food choices which help heal the body naturally verses the powerful chemicals found in highly processed, manufactured, and refined foods.

It uses technology that reads your body's nutrient and hormonal imbalances similar to how an EEG, EKG, or MRI scans for their specific purposes.

The NRF (NutriMost Resonant Frequency) cell scanning technology essentially takes your hormonal fingerprint to determine the exact ingredients you need to bring your body into an optimal state of fat burning and resets your metabolism to keep the weight off. The results provide a picture of what foods work for you and which ones contribute to weight gain.

No two people are the same. You'll learn what foods to eat and which to avoid that are unique to you. The other diet plans are generalized as to what is good or not good to eat, but this plan scientifically determines exactly how the foods affect your ability to burn fat and regain your health. It's not the foods themselves that are "bad." But they may not be right for you,

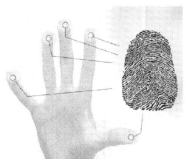

and without the scanning process you may never discover it.

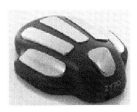

Because of this scanning process, each person gets an individualized plan which includes a specific list of foods and supplements to use during the initial 40 days of the diet. One of the keys to this plan is alkaline water and the high pH factor. Energy sapping sugar and oil are restricted for the first 40 days.

It requires no drugs or hormones, no pre-packaged meals, and no exercise during the diet phase. Increased energy throughout the plan is common.

Your metabolic age is tracked as well as your body fat level, hydration, visceral fat rating, BMI and more. It's not uncommon to go from an unhealthy metabolic age to a much younger age. This number comes from comparing all the body factors, including percentage of body fat and water, muscle mass and Basal Metabolic Rate compared with the average of your chronological age group. A low metabolic age indicates a fast metabolism making it very easy to lose weight and maintain your weight. A high metabolic age indicates you have slow metabolism with weight loss resistance and exercise resistance. It's a great goal to have your metabolic age much lower than your actual age.

Another important number is your visceral fat rating. This is the fat in the abdominal cavity surrounding your vital organs. Aging causes the fat to shift into the abdominal area (belly fat!)

and can cause health issues. It's best to have a visceral fat rating below 12.

Diabetic patients are required to monitor their blood sugar daily and work closely with their NutriMost doctor. This is the plan that my husband chose. Within a couple of weeks on the plan, and daily reporting with his NutriMost doctor, he shared his progress with his primary doctor, who eliminated his most harmful long-term diabetic prescription. He no longer needed it to control his blood sugar levels. **Given the proper foods, the body can heal itself.**

The results can be permanent because it addresses the cause of your weight problem. Once your metabolism is reset, you should be able to maintain the new, healthier weight.

There is another diet (hCG based) that is somewhat similar on the surface. I do not recommend this. It singularly focuses on rapid weight loss, but does not have any of the scanning or supplementation controls of NutriMost. The dieter is left to determine his own food choices and "sensible" meals.

Unfortunately, what is sensible to one might not be to another, and some are not even close to what's best. It may use generic synthetic hormone drops or pills. They aren't adjusted to the dieter's needs. This means no assurance of getting the proper nutrition as the fat burns off. There is no control of electrolytes, glucose or antioxidant protection, all part of the NutriMost plan.

In contrast to that, the creator of NutriMost, Dr. Ray Wisniewski, has received numerous awards and accolades for Clinical Excellence and outstanding excellence in patient care.

To learn more about NutriMost or find a doctor near you, visit NutriMost.com. If you're in the Dallas, TX. area, I recommend Dr. George at burnfatdfw.com.

## Sugar and Carbohydrates

To stay in a healthy range, a person should not have more than 32 grams (8 teaspoons) of added sugar per day. This is especially true if you're already overweight or have blood sugar problems.

There are different types of sugar and they are hidden everywhere. Many people fail to realize the amount of sugar that's hidden in the carbohydrates they consume each day.

Soda and energy drinks account for over 35% of American's added sugars. Eliminating or restricting them is a good start.

Refined, processed carbohydrates are very dangerous and you should always try to avoid them, especially white bread, white pasta, white potatoes, or white rice. These types of foods are VERY high in the glycemic index and will cause your blood sugar to spike, which then causes your pancreas to work very hard to produce insulin trying to regulate your blood sugar.

Because they cause a spike your blood sugar, these foods will typically make you hungry again much quicker.

## FREE FOODS IN A DIABETIC DIET

Even when there are free foods on a diabetic diet, it doesn't mean you don't have to pay for them. What it does mean is you can eat them freely without considering them an exchange or counting them as carbohydrates. These are the kinds of foods that you are going to want around the house in abundance for times when you're hungry and meal time is still too far away.

Free foods have little to no affect on blood sugars and that's why they can be eaten without counting them as part of a meal. Your doctor or dietician will provide you with a complete list, but here are a few items that are normally considered free foods:

* Water (alkaline water with a pH of 8.5-9.5 is best) and other water-based drinks that are sugar free (limit coffee and tea use)
* Bouillon (beef, chicken, or vegetable broth). This is high sodium so use in balance with other foods
* Sugar-free gelatin (flavored or not)
* Pickles
* Cream Cheese
* Unsweetened cocoa powder
* Rhubarb

* Cranberries

* Salsa

Many condiments are considered free foods too. When you're planning a snack or a meal add some of the free foods such as salsa or a small amount of cream cheese for variety or extra flavor. Skip the mayo!

Also, add cinnamon daily (capsules or ½ tsp on foods). It helps lower blood sugar and is good for the heart.

Depending on your dietician, he or she may consider most vegetables as part of the free foods group too. Vegetables that do not qualify include potatoes, corn, peas, and carrots as they are considered starchy and have higher carbohydrate content. If your dietician does allow you to have vegetables in between meals, make sure to clarify which ones and in what quantities.

## SAFE DIABETIC FOOD OPTIONS

Your mind may be swimming with all this information. From breakfast to bedtime, just what are some safe food options? Here's a short list to get you started. I'm grouping the foods for you from morning to evening with snacks in the mix to help you get started. Some are meals, some are foods to combine to create your meals. Mix and match, use your imagination.

Oatmeal with nuts and fruit

Burrito - scrambled eggs, onions, peppers, black beans, salsa, cheese, whole grain tortilla

Cottage cheese and fresh fruit

Power smoothie (fruits, veggies, protein powder, whatever you want it to be)

Hard boiled eggs and cheese

Whole grain cereal, including the bran, no sugars

Turkey or chicken (not processed lunch meat) layered on whole grain bread, tomato, and Avocado

Lean chicken, Canadian bacon, turkey sausage, salmon

Fresh or fresh frozen and yogurt

Unsweetened pomegranate juice

Range free eggs, omega 3 fortified

Low fat yogurt (Greek is best)

Healthy dairy products

Veggie scramble, black beans and cheese

Pair fruits with nuts, cheeses

Nuts, seeds, some soy foods

Grass fed, high quality meats

French cheeses, or American if from grass fed cows

Homemade baked potato skins with cheese

Thin turkey slice with veggies

Plain popcorn, air popped

Celery sticks with cream cheese or peanut butter

Veggies and cheese (not processed)

Dips from yogurt and diced cucumbers, etc. with veggie sticks

Eat salads, veggies, beans, salmon, hard boiled eggs

Coffee - black, regular or decaf (one-two cups max per day)

Tea (green, black, red)

Beans- diabetic super food

Bananas (not over ripe)

Properly prepared potatoes and yams

**64 oz of water daily** - for variety add fruit or veggie slices to pitcher. Water with fresh lemons; unsweetened pomegranate or blueberry juice; moderate use of diet Soda Stream mixes; DON'T mix with powdered packaged flavorings. Try high alkaline, pH balanced water.

**Fish** – deep sea, cold water fish; Pacific wild salmon (better than Atlantic salmon); tuna, halibut, rainbow trout and scallops

**Healing vegetables**: 3-5 servings per day, raw are best - Salads (dark greens like Romaine are better than iceberg); lightly steamed; raw veggie snacks; fresh vegetable juice; mashed potato and cauliflower combination; slaw mixed with oil and vinegar

**Hearty whole grains** – hot cereals, especially oatmeal; slow cooking, nothing instant; Ezekiel breads, sprouted grain; unsweetened homemade granola; add fruits, cinnamon; whole grain pasta (Racconto); rye, barley, quinoa, spelt, whole wheat; buckwheat, oats, brown rice, millet, limited corn.

Many diets refer to fruits and vegetables being wise for anyone's diet. However, many fruits are high in natural sugars. You may want to limit your consumption of fruits and juices such as oranges, apples, and pineapple until you have a handle on your blood sugar numbers. Also, pure fruit juice is far superior to watered down fruit drinks which have less nutritional value and are higher in sugar.

Some foods may react differently depending on your blood type. If you find that you have adverse reactions to certain foods such as consistent upset stomach or draggy, lethargic feeling after eating, you might want to check out information about the blood type diet. According to the blood type diet, a person with O blood type does well with animal proteins while the A, B, and AB blood types do better with vegetarian foods. This is a generalization, but something you may want to be aware of.

# SECTION 3 – WHEN TO EAT, ADAPTING DIETS, READING LABELS, AND MORE

## WHEN TO EAT WHEN YOU HAVE DIABETES

As a diabetic when you eat may be just as important as what you eat. Keeping a steady stream of food in your system without causing high blood sugars can be hard to do. But once you figure what works for you, you will have more flexibility and better control of your diabetes.

It is recommended that diabetics eat many small meals throughout the day or three main meals and three snacks in between. A typical day may go like this:

* Wake-up and have breakfast
* Mid-morning snack
* Lunch
* Mid-afternoon snack
* Dinner
* Bedtime snack

The timing in between each meal or snack should be two to three hours. This variation will depend on what you have eaten at the previous meal, how active you have been and how you feel.    If you're feeling hungry or light-headed and you normally wouldn't have eaten for another 30 minutes, don't wait. Test your blood sugar and move up your meal. The time it can take for you to wait the 30 minutes can be the time it takes for your blood sugar to drop dangerously low.

The only time you may want to wait a longer period of time is between dinner and your bedtime snack. Most times dinner is the biggest meal of the day and you will not need food again for a longer period of time. Another reason to wait longer is to ensure that you have enough food in your system before you go to bed to last you through the night without your blood sugars dropping too low.

If alternating meals and snacks doesn't work for you, consider eating smaller meals and smaller portion sizes. Eating this way (less more often) makes it easier for your body to regulate blood glucose levels.

## ADJUSTING YOUR DIABETIC DIET FOR SPECIAL OCCASIONS

Birthdays, Halloween, Thanksgiving, Christmas, and other holidays and special occasions are often centered around food. For most people these are times to anticipate the celebration and the eating.

Unfortunately, much of the foods are the opposite of what is healthy for a diabetic. It doesn't have to be a stressful time if you anticipate the occasions and decide how you wish to adapt your eating.

The hardest part may be not knowing what is going to be served. If this is the case, a quick call to your host or hostess can help. Most people a happy to accommodate their guests' dietary needs. Then plan your meals for that day accordingly. You may want to have fewer carbohydrates with your breakfast and snack to make up for the extra ones you will have at a birthday party where pizza is being served. And still limit the quantities of your celebration meals.

Another option for special occasions is to offer to bring a dish for everyone to share. Make it something that you enjoy as a treat but still follows the guidelines for your diabetic diet.

For family favorites and traditions, be creative and look for ways to make the same dishes with less fat or sugar. You can do this by substituting a sugar substitute like Stevia for regular sugar, or choose whole wheat flour instead of white for the extra fiber content.

During the holidays and other occasions, closely monitor your blood sugars. Even with extra care, the change in your diet can still result in a blood sugar that is too high or low.

## SNACKING ON NUTS – MORE HEALTHY THAN YOU THOUGHT

Eating a handful of nuts 4 to 5 times a week lowers risks of heart related problems and can contribute to weight loss. That has been proved by several studies that were conducted to research the nutritional values. Nuts are good sources of different minerals and nutrients and are important for living a disease-free life.

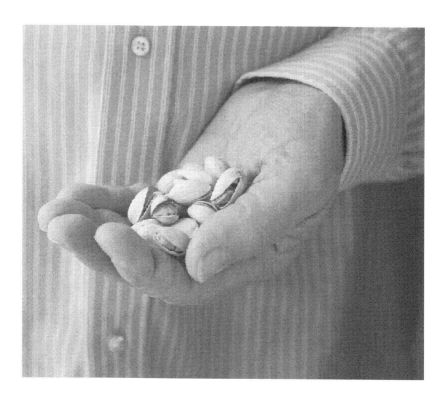

Health benefits come from the mono and polyunsaturated fat found in nuts. They can increase the level of good cholesterol in the body. Nuts are also good providers of thiamin, niacin, phosphorous, zinc, folate, selenium, copper, magnesium, manganese, potassium, iron, and vitamin E. These nutrients can be found in certain types of nuts.

Almonds are a good source of iron, magnesium, zinc, and vitamin E. Sweet almonds are the ones being eaten while bitter almonds serve as oil. Selenium, which helps prevent prostate cancer and is important for the proper functioning of the thyroid gland, can be found in Brazil nuts. Cashews serve as a good source of copper that aids to lower blood pressure. If you are interested in the type of nut that contains the lowest amount of fat, you are looking for chestnuts. Chestnuts only get 8% of their calorie content from fat unlike most nuts which get 75% of calorie from fat.

Hazelnuts alternatively provide 80% of the recommended daily allowance of manganese in just a handful. Along with hazelnuts, Macadamia nuts provide manganese which helps in the production of sex hormones and is necessary for healthy skin, bones, and joints.

Peanuts, which are not actually nuts but legumes, help in the formation of nitric oxide, a substance that widens arteries including those which supply blood to the genital area resulting to a man's sexual wellness. Peanuts have the potential of helping people lose weight because they contain high fiber, protein, and fat content. Studies from Purdue and Harvard compared peanuts with other low-fat snacks such as rice cakes, and the results showed that peanuts can keep us from hunger for two hours unlike the latter which only worked for half an hour.

Walnuts are tested to have high levels of omega-3 fatty acids like alphalinolenic acid (ALA) which helps prevent abnormal heart rhythms that usually lead to heart attack or worse, sudden cardiac death.

But, of course, these benefits will only work if they are consumed in proper quantity. Over do it and the effect will be the exact opposite.

Experts only suggest a handful of nuts 4 to 5 times a week. A handful means 22 almonds, 18 cashews, 12 macadamia nuts, 14 walnut halves, 7 Brazil nuts, 20 hazelnuts or 28 peanuts. Eat nuts toasted or roasted without salt and not fried with hydrogenated fat. Keep large quantities of nuts in an air-tight container in your freezer. They have a very long shelf life and can be stored for six months.

## HIGH FAT FOODS AND THEIR EFFECT ON BLOOD SUGAR

All diets should use fat in moderation as it can lead to an unhealthy body weight and heart disease. For a diabetic, controlling fat intake is important for these reasons in addition to the negative effect it can have on blood sugars. Fats can be put into many different categories: healthy, non-healthy, saturated, non-saturated, trans-fat, and more. But the bottom line with any of kind of fat is to enjoy it in moderation.

When you eat food that is high in fat (for instance a cheeseburger), your short-term blood glucose reading may come back as fine. But since fat acts much like protein and it slows down the digestion of carbohydrates, you may notice a higher than normal blood sugar many hours later. It's hard to plan for such a spike because it is quite delayed compared to other foods that quickly raise blood sugar.

The best advice is to choose natural, healthy, unsaturated fats and oils whenever possible. You can do this by reading your food labels carefully as the different kinds of fats are listed on most food labels. Excessive fat intake will also cause you to gain weight and that is another way blood sugars can spiral out of control. Extra body weight that you carry around is taxing on your systems and will affect how your body uses and needs insulin. Your visceral fat (the fat around your organs) should be no higher than 12.

Healthy fat choices include:

* Avocado – oil or the fruit itself
* Coconut oil
* Sesame or olive oil
* Black or green olives
* Peanuts and peanut butter (this doubles as a protein choice)
* Sesame seeds

Additional fat choices that should be used in moderation:

* Butter (Choose butter instead of margarine)
* Walnuts
* Salad dressings
* Mayonnaise
* Pumpkin and sunflower seeds

Unprocessed coconut oil and avocado oil are heart healthy oils. Coconut in all forms helps with metabolism and fat loss. Use coconut or avocado oil in place of other oils, including olive oil. There are reports that several brands of olive oil have added non-olive oil, such as canola oil.

Avocado oil is good for cooking because it has a high burn temperature. Coconut oil doesn't need to be refrigerated and has a low melt temperature. It has a wide variety of healthy uses.

If you have questions about a type of fat and what a serving size should be, contact your doctor or dietician for more information.

## WHEN YOU ARE HUNGRY IN BETWEEN MEALS

There will be times when you've finished your meal or snack and you're hungry again long before your next meal is scheduled, or right before bed. Depending on how much time you have before you're supposed to eat again, as well as what your blood sugar levels are, you may want to move your meal time up or indulge in some free food.

If this happens frequently it's time to look at your eating schedule and meal plan. If you've recently added more physical activity to your daily routine, you may have to increase your food intake to compensate for the extra energy you're using up. If this isn't the case, and you're unsure why your appetite has increased or your current meal plan is no longer working, speak to your dietician to see if there are some revisions that can be made to prevent this from continuing.

When you have gestational diabetes, it is recommended that you have a snack before bedtime to tide you over until the morning. It will also be important to have a bedtime snack if you are taking an insulin injection prior to bed so that your blood sugar does not become too low overnight.

If neither of these scenarios applies to you, you can have some free food before bed if you're hungry at night. A bouillon (beef, vegetable, or chicken broth) might stave off hunger pangs and allow you to fall asleep.

If you're hungry at night time and your blood sugars are low, do have something to eat to raise your glucose level. If this is a frequent occurrence, you may not be eating enough food at dinner time. Try adding a protein or healthy carbohydrate to see if this makes a difference.

## ARTIFICIAL SWEETENERS MAY NOT BE SO SWEET

The food industry came up with what they thought was a solution for people on diets or with diabetes and a sweet tooth. Artificial sweeteners are used in everything from chewing gum, coffee sweeteners, sodas, and baking. Controversy over their use exists over real health benefits or the negative affect they can cause to the unsuspecting consumer. Some artificial sweeteners are synthetic and others are derived from the actual sugar plant.

The four different kinds of artificial sweeteners are: saccharin, aspartame, sucralose, and acesulfame potassium. Each of these types can be found under various product names and brands. Not all are made the same way and they have different uses. Some you can buy in liquid or powdered form for baking needs and others, like aspartame, is only found in foods that you purchase pre-made.

While the use of these artificial sweeteners will not raise blood sugar, the food items with these artificial sweeteners will still have an effect on your blood sugar. Aspartame has been linked in some medical studies with Alzheimer's disease. It's also been linked to increased cravings for carbohydrates. Studies show those who drink diet sodas often gain weight.

Some diabetics prefer to use honey as a substitute for sugar. However, honey is very similar to sugar in carbohydrate content and the effects it will have on your blood glucose level. It is best to enjoy honey in small amounts, if at all. Local raw honey, if available, is best because it minimizes allergy responses.

Stevia, on the other hand, is a plant that is a natural sweetener without the negative effects of the commercially made artificial sweeteners and is a better choice for your health. Chemically manufactured foods generally do not have positive health benefits, and when you have diabetes, you should eat as much natural and healthy foods as possible, including your choice of sweeteners.

## READING FOOD LABELS

Reading food labels seems to be the most effective way of determining the right kind of food to be bought in the supermarket. It lets you make sensible food selections. The food label includes important information to a diabetic. Learning to read them and understanding the numbers and percentages will help you make wise food choices.

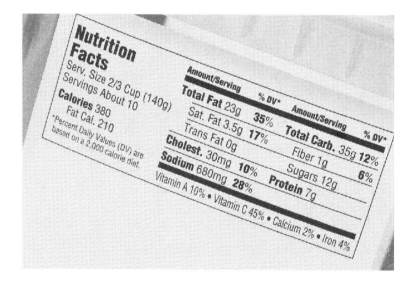

Whether you're counting carbohydrates, following a specific diet, or just trying to properly balance what you eat, you'll increase your chances for success by reading your food labels and understanding what they mean.

The ingredient list is a good place to start before looking at the numbers in the food label. Ingredients are listed in order of quantity to the entire product. If sugar is listed first, there is more sugar in that product than anything else. The closer it is to the beginning of the list the more of it is present in the food. Avoid foods that list items that don't work well for you. Products with a lot of unpronounceable chemical ingredients should be avoided too.

Look at the serving size and compare that to the number of carbohydrates in a serving. Diabetic serving size for carbohydrates is usually 15 grams. If one serving is higher than 15 grams, you'll have to eat less than the suggested serving size to stay on track with your meal plan.

Sugar-free foods may grab your attention as something safe and yummy to add to your shopping cart. But look at the carbohydrate count first. Most foods that are made sugar-free using artificial sweeteners and sugar substitutes have higher carbohydrate counts. Often fat is increased to compensate the flavor when limiting or removing sugar. There are always tradeoffs to make the foods taste better.

Check the fat content too. Look for a low percent of your daily intake and ideally it will be monounsaturated, as opposed to polyunsaturated or saturated fats.

**Be prepared to put things back on the shelves.**

Through the "Nutrition Facts" section of the label, you can identify the amount of serving sizes provided in that product. You can clearly understand the amount and kinds of nutrients that are included. Usually, the label contains the information on saturated fat, sodium, total fat, fiber, and cholesterol amount "per serving," based on a 2000 calorie diet.

Here's a list of things that you need to know:

**Serving size**

The amount of servings stated in the food label refers to the quantity of food people usually consume. However, this does not necessarily mean that it reflects your very own amount of food intake.

Moreover, serving size determines the amount of nutrients that enter the body. This means that if you will follow strictly what the serving size is, you will obtain the same amount of nutrients according to the serving size that was given in the label.

We live in a supersized world, and most people are surprised to find that their idea of a restaurant meal single serving is actually two or three servings. So, we've gotten used to larger quantities.

In some cases, in order to get you to buy a product that's high in fat or sugar or carbs, the manufacturer cleverly shows acceptable amounts but increases the number of servings. Or it might be that you consume the entire package even though it clearly shows it the "family size." Therefore, if it's something you eat in a single serving but shows 3 servings, multiply the number of servings by the grams/calories shown to get the real amounts and their effect on your body. Ouch!

**Nutrients**

This refers to the list of available nutrients in a particular item. It's also where the nutritional claims of the product based on the recommended daily dietary allowance are stated. Usually, the nutritional amounts are based on recommended 2,000-2,500 calorie dietary allowances.

In order to understand the numeric value of each item, you should know that the "% daily value" that the food label indicates is based on how a food corresponds to the recommended daily dietary allowance for 2,000 calories eaten in a day.

If you have a monitoring system, such as Fitbit or the other wearables, you may be able to see how many calories you are consuming in a 24-hour period. If you're a small female, for example, you may be gaining weight if you consume over 1500 calories in a day! It won't take much of an indulgence to throw you off course. Awareness helps.

**Label claim**

This refers to the kinds of nutritional claims of a food item. For instance, if an item says it is sodium-free, it has less than 5 milligrams per serving or a low-fat item may contain 3 grams of fat or less.

Indeed, reading food labels can be very tedious and confusing at first. Nevertheless, once you get the hang of it, it will be easier for you to maintain your diet because you can control the amount of foods that you take in.

## TIPS FOR REVAMPING RECIPES

Everyone has their favorite dishes, ones that mom or grandma used to make, or new ones that you have discovered on your own. Once diagnosed with diabetes, you may feel that you can never enjoy these dishes again (or not without harming your health). But there are ways that you can change old family favorites, keeping the flavor but reducing or eliminating the amount of sugar or carbohydrates they contain.

For most substitutions that you're going to make to your recipes, you're looking for ways to reduce the fat content. Here are some standards that you can use. When your recipe calls for

* Whole milk, try substituting with 2% or 1% instead
* Whole eggs, try using an egg substitute or use 2 egg whites for every whole egg called for
* Sour cream, use low fat sour cream or plain yogurt
* Baking chocolate, try using cocoa powder mixed with coconut oil (3 tablespoons with 1 tablespoon of oil will equal 1 ounce of chocolate)

In addition to the above suggestions, always use light or lower fat versions of ingredients. Sometimes trial and error is necessary to get the recipe just right, but do keep trying. The result will be worth it when you create a cake or other dessert that you love and it's now diabetic friendly.

Alternately, you can purchase a diabetic cook book that is full of tasty meals and desserts that will work with your diet. This way you can create new favorites for you and your family to fall in love with. Don't feel that you can't enjoy variety in your foods. Keep trying new things while keeping a close eye on your blood sugar levels as you add new foods to your growing repertoire.

## MEAL PLANNING FOR ACTIVE DIABETICS

Physical activity is recommended for any person to stay healthy. But for a diabetic it not only increases energy levels and helps maintain an ideal body weight, it also helps to control blood sugars. But an active diabetic needs to take extra care and precautions to ensure getting enough fuel so blood sugar levels don't drop dangerously low, known as hypoglycemia.

The amount you exercise is going to determine how much you are going to eat on your diabetic meal plan. The more physically active you are the higher your nutritional requirements and the higher your risk is for developing hypoglycemia. The best practice when you are just starting out is to monitor your blood sugars before and after working out and during if you feel it is necessary. It is important to listen to your body and stop if you are feeling light-headed or are experiencing any of the other signs associated with low blood sugar.

Before you work out, have a snack that is going to sustain you for a long period of time without spiking your blood sugar levels. A granola bar eaten with a handful of nuts is a good choice as it combines a carbohydrate that is high in fiber and a high-quality protein. The food that you eat before working out should have high fiber content, as this will slow down the process of carbohydrates in your system. You will be sustained for a longer period of time.

Drink plenty of fluids (preferably water) to stay hydrated when you're working out. In case of an emergency, carry glucose tablets with you or some hard candy that will quickly raise your blood sugar. At other times of the day, eat balanced meals to maintain your energy.

## EASY MEAL PLANNING

Meal planning is essential to a successful diabetic diet. It will prevent times when you don't have anything ready for dinner and grab something that you probably shouldn't be eating. The planning should begin before you head to the grocery store so you know what ingredients you need. You'll be less tempted to stray from your diet plans.

Once a week, sit down and plan what meals you're going to eat for the next week. Or you could do this for a month at a time. When making your meal plan, don't forget to include all meals and snacks too. If you're hungry and know what and when your next meal is going to be, you are going to be better prepared.

In the beginning, meal planning will take some time. Depending on which diet you're following, you're going to need to get used to the foods you can have, the portion sizes and how they can be cooked.

Plan each day out in its entirety. Make it realistic; don't plan to make vegetable lasagna on a night that you know you won't be home until late. Save the meals with more preparation for when you have time and make extra so you can have leftovers.

Don't go to the grocery store when you're hungry. If you do, there's more chance that you'll buy foods that you don't need or that are unhealthy. Another trick while you're pushing the cart around is to only get what is on your list. This will help you stick to your meal plan and can save you money too.

## STAYING ON TRACK

Once you've taken the time to plan your meals and snacks for the week and have gone grocery shopping, you're all set for a week's worth of healthy eating. Sometimes the best plans can go astray. You also need to know how to get back on track and stay motivated to follow your diabetic diet.

For some, staying on track is relatively easy. Their motivation is high. For others, they may need more variety or just better understanding of the health benefits and consequences of not eating per their diabetic needs. Saying "it's not fair" doesn't help much.

If that's you, you might try doing some research or talking to other diabetics and your dietician for suggestions on how to mix up your eating plan.

If you're the only person in your family with diabetes, encourage others to support your efforts. Ask them to join you in the healthier meals, or at least not eat things in front of you that you can't have. Working together on recipes or meal planning can result in closer family ties.

If you're feeling alone and a bit resentful that you can't eat what and when you want, then consider joining a support group for diabetics. Not only can they help you through the times you want to cheat on your diet, they can also provide emotional support. Talking to others who have been through the same thing will help and encourage you to stay on your meal plan for the right reasons.

Sometimes money can be a factor. Higher quality foods can be more expensive than the quick and easy convenience foods. Try easing the better foods into your diet as much as possible. Cutting out the desserts and unwise snacks can save money as well. You may discover that you can reduce or eliminate some of your medications which creates an even bigger money savings.

# SECTION 4 - EXERCISE AND DIABETES

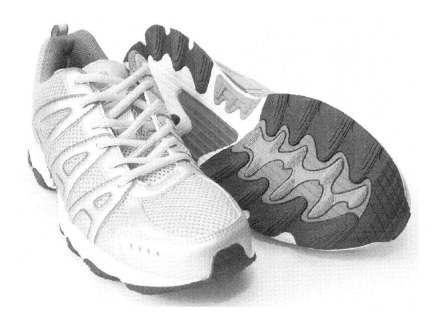

One of the most undemanding and workable ways to regulate blood sugar, eliminate the dangers of "cardiovascular disease," and perk up health and welfare in general is exercise.

We live in an inactive world where many jobs are managed from an ergonomic chair in front of a computer. Electronic games and social media keep people tied to computers and mobile devices. Exercise can come last in your day's event planning.

## THE WEIGHT OF EXERCISE

Everyone should exercise, yet only 30% of the United States population gets the recommended thirty minutes of daily physical activity, and 25% are not active at all. In fact, inactivity is thought to be one of the key reasons for the surge of type 2 diabetes in the U.S. Inactivity and obesity promote insulin resistance.

The good news is that it's never too late to get moving, and exercise is one of the easiest ways to start controlling your diabetes. Especially for people with type 2 diabetes, exercise can improve insulin sensitivity, lower the risk of heart disease, and promote weight loss.

Without exercise, people have the tendency to become obese. Once they are obese, they have bigger chances of accumulating type 2 diabetes or complications from it.

Today, the U.S. Department of Health and Human Services reports that over 80% of people with type 2 diabetes are clinically overweight. It's time to start doing those jumping and stretching activities.

## GETTING STARTED

The first order of business with any exercise plan, especially if you are "dyed-in-the-wool" sluggish, is to consult with your health care provider. If you have cardiac risk factors, the health care provider may want to perform a stress test to establish a safe level of exercise for you.

Certain diabetic complications will also dictate what type of exercise program you can take on. Activities like weightlifting, jogging, or high-impact aerobics can possibly pose a risk for people with diabetic retinopathy due to the risk for further blood vessel damage and possible retinal detachment.

If you are already active in sports or work out regularly, it will still benefit you to discuss your regular routine with your doctor. If you are taking insulin, you may need to take special precautions to prevent hypoglycemia during your workout.

## START SLOW

One of the easiest and least expensive ways of getting moving is to start a walking program. All you need is a good pair of well-fitting, supportive shoes and a direction to head in.

Your exercise routine can be as simple as a brisk nightly neighborhood walk. If you haven't been very active before now, start slowly and work your way up. Walk the dog or get out in the yard and rake leaves. Take the stairs instead of the elevator. Park in the back of the lot and walk. Every little bit works. In fact, it helps a lot.

As little as 15 to 30 minutes of daily, heart-pumping exercise can make a big difference in your blood glucose control and your risk of developing diabetic complications. Ramp it up as you get used to the routine and your health care provider says it's ok.

You don't have to invest in costly health club memberships, or the most up-to-date health device to start pumping those fats out. What you need is the willingness and the determination to start exercising to a healthier lifestyle.

# CONCLUSION AND NEXT STEPS

**Life is a journey, not a destination.**  I know that the most important step is the decision to make changes, however small. You went through life experiences, good and bad, and made it to today. Now you can choose to smooth out the bumps, aim for a better, higher destination. It's never a straight line to the top, but by making small corrections along the way, you can have a smoother ride from now on.

**How many years to do you *want* to live?**  Don't look at today's conditions to determine that number, but look into your heart.  How big is that number? There are no wrong answers here. Mine is 120! Next, *imagine yourself on your last birthday, celebrating that you have arrived at that year*. Where would you be celebrating?  Who would be with you? Imagine the scene in as great a detail as you can.

I hope you smiled as you thought of your victories, and of what might be possible. Hold that positive image in your mind's eye, and then think through your present situation.

What changes need to be made so you can arrive at that birthday celebration? You've no doubt heard the expression "You're only as old as you feel." Some of us feel old when

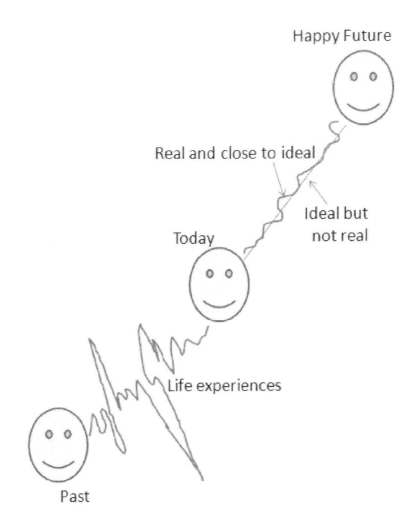

we're relatively young. Others choose to feel young on purpose. I encourage you to be part of that group!

Keep making the corrections along the path. Catch the dips before they become slides. Keep the destination of good health fixed in your mind. Share your destination and healthy life with someone if you wish. Plan your path, prepare the supplies, and blast off to a great future!

**Another exercise to lock in your reasons to commit** to a healthier lifestyle involves a bit of thought, and is well worth it. *Write out what value you bring to yourself and those around you,* including all the roles you have – parent, income earner, child, friend, coach, employee, employer, etc. You get the picture. *Now write out another list of what you and everyone else would lose out on if you don't take care of yourself,* even to the point of you becoming blind or having any of the seriously negative things happen. It's okay to be dramatic here. It's not ego, and it's not the time to think nobody would care – trust me, they do!

You might discover you're much more valuable that you give yourself credit for (remember George Bailey in *It's a Wonderful Life*). You have many people counting on you and what your unique gifts bring to others. Writing out the worst things that could happen if you aren't in the picture anymore can give you a boost when you're tempted to give up or give in to those temptations.

Everyone has a unique 1% that he or she brings to the world. What's yours? If you'd like to find out more information about how to discover your unique value, email me at Marian@SuccessPerspectives.com with your thoughts or questions. I will reply personally.

I wish you the healthiest lifestyle possible! It is YOUR choice! Listen to your physician, but be proactive in your own diabetic cure.

# COMPANION JOURNAL

Look for the companion *Diabetes Journal*. It's a place where you can collect your health tips and favorite recipes in one place. Keep your Food Diary here.

Track progress. Enter weight, moods, health concerns and successes. Make notes about what foods work well with your body, and what foods are negative triggers.

See something delicious and diabetes-friendly on Facebook? Jot it in your *Diabetes Journal*.

Converted a family favorite recipe? Record it in the book so you can make it the same way again.

A good progress report? Add that to your *Diabetes Journal,* too, so you can stay motivated. Add in Before and After pictures. And whatever else you can think of!

Enjoy the process. You're worth it!

# ABOUT THE AUTHOR

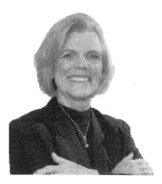

Marian Hays writes on a variety of subjects with the aim of inspiring others how to get unstuck and take action to discover their own positive results.

A lifelong reader and researcher, she's shared her findings with anyone who was interested (and sometimes just someone within earshot). Encouraged by others to share her information and insights with a broader audience, she's now reaching out through books, articles, audio, video trainings and more.

She lives in the Dallas, Texas, area with her husband and their cat. Visit her website at SuccessPerspectives.com.

## PUBLISHERS NOTES

### DISCLAIMER

This publication is intended to provide helpful and informative material. It is not intended to diagnose, treat, cure, or prevent any health problem or condition, nor is intended to replace the advice of a physician. No action should be taken solely on the contents of this book. Always consult your physician or qualified health-care professional on any matters regarding your health and before adopting any suggestions in this book or drawing inferences from it.

The author and publisher specifically disclaim all responsibility for any liability, loss, or risk, personal or otherwise, which is incurred as a consequence, directly or indirectly, from the use or application of any contents of this book.

Any and all product names referenced within this book are the trademarks of their respective owners. None of these owners have sponsored, authorized, endorsed, or approved this book.

Always read all information provided by the manufacturers' product labels before using their products. The author and publisher are not responsible for claims made by manufacturers.

If expert advice or assistance is required, the services of a competent professional person should be sought.

## REVISED EDITION

This book has been updated from the original Kindle publication, *Diabetes Diet Options – What to Eat, When to Eat and How to Regain Your Health,* published in 2013. New cover, new content added.

Manufactured in the United States of America

## YOUR REVIEWS

If you found this book to be helpful, please leave a review at the book's page on Amazon.com. You'll help others in the process, and the author will be very grateful. Thanks!

Marian Hays

118

Made in the USA
San Bernardino, CA
09 January 2017